BADASS BODY DIET
6 WEEKS SLIM DOWN
Weight Loss Challenge

Burn Fat and Boost Metabolism Fast Forever

by Changing Life Habits

You are a badass

By
WaraWaran Roongruangsri

Author's Note

Most people know how to exercise and eat well. It is more important to maximize that knowledge and moreover fine tuning it. This should be done so that you can achieve great results in record time. We often tend to overlook the minor details. Although we all aware of the facts and methods but we still overlook them and cheat on our own plans.

Becoming fit requires discipline and hard work, but seven weeks of both can transform your body into something that looks and feels great. You've got the information right in front of you. I have seen this method work again and again, for all ages. It has worked for both men and women. All it requires is your sincere efforts and your heart.

So are you ready to step away and break the unhealthy lifestyle trend?

Introducing "Badass Body Diet 6 Weeks Slim Down"

This powerful guide will provide you with all the vital ingredients that you need for quick and effective results. These are not myths or miraculous cures, these are simple truths that we know but we often overlook and do not follow it in a daily routine.

When you grab this guide and incorporate it into your life you will be well on your way to shedding the extra pounds so that you can become stronger and fitter than ever.

Weight loss promises are the ones that you make to yourself all day and night, but the hard part is actually keeping those promises to yourself.

With the help of this guide you will discover information about the following:-

- Learn The Proper Steps To Maximize Results
- Discover The Truth On Food Labels
- Quickly Get Results By Incorporating The Right Type Of Cardio
- Nutrition Overhaul

Thanks again for downloading this book, I hope you enjoy it!

WaraWaran Roongruangsri

Table of Contents

INTRODUCTION

The new statistics and study of the food facts around the globe suggest that the people in the world are suffering more from obesity than from starvation. Now, that is a startling fact. All this while, it was certainly believed that starvation is a bigger problem to deal with. But now dealing with obesity has drawn more attention.An estimate shows the number of obese is 1 billion as compared to 800 million people who are not fed properly.

It is definitely not a surprising fact that the most affected parts of the world are the mostly the western countries. The United States, Western Europe, Canada and Australia are the worst affected countries of the world. In order to control this condition one has to be very careful. When one eats the same diet every day and leads an inactive life, this affects your metabolism directly. Ultimately not paying attention to your diet will tend to result in an unhealthy lifestyle. An unhealthy lifestyle will affect you in a lot of ways. The most important conclusion out of an unhealthy lifestyle is that it will make the quality of your life low.

There are two main reasons why the world is getting fat and why is the whole world experiencing the obesity epidemic. Although it is not at all hard to guess that all the reasons are well worth exploring.

We have adopted certain lifestyle trends worldwide. It would not be wrong to say that we have adopted certain trends related to diet surprisingly in the whole world. It has now become very important to find the root of these trends and break them. We can bring perfect peace and attain balance into our life by just altering the wrong trends related to lifestyle and diet that we have developed during the recent years. We all want to look good and feel healthy. And nobody but we shall have to work to achieve that.

It is perfectly dependent upon you if you want to become the person who is fat and unhealthy or who is healthy and not sick.Becoming fit requires discipline and hard work, but six weeks of both can transform your body into what looks attractive and feels great. You have got the information right in front of you. I have seen this method work again and again, for all age groups. It has worked for women and men both. It only requires your sincere efforts and your heart. Nobody but you will be solely responsible for this transformation. All you have to do is maintain your focus on achieving a healthy diet.

You have already committed and got yourself a copy of our Badass Body Diet, a 6 week slim down challenge for weight loss. The next two very important and rather challenging steps would be to read the guide and follow the instructions properly. Well, I have faith that you will succeed in acting upon these instructions because you ae committed towards achieving your goal.

So, what are you waiting for! So a lifetime of a healthy lifestyle and dynamic vibrant looks is waiting for you. Make absolutely no mistakesand you can definitely do it.

Let us get started!

GET READY TO BEGIN BADASS BODY DIET 6 WEEK SLIM DOWN

Before we understand about the "how to do" and "why to do" of our Badass Body Diet 6 Weeks Slim Down there are two things that we will cover which will help you achieve all your fitness dreams. Even the wildest ones! These are basically x-factors which are often skipped in other weigh loss programs and they are not conveyed to you by the fitness instructors as well. You should not be making any mistake in grasping them as these factors are absolute game changers. These are 100% tried and tested. These are the factors that are enough to motivate you in your worst times even.

The 1st will besetting a realistic goal for yourself. The second is concrete advice on choosing the right kind of training partner for yourself. You must be very sure about these two, because throughout your 6 week slim down they prove to be the most crucial factors while you achieve your goal.

Setting a SMART Realistic Fitness Goal

The ultimate result of your hard work will depend upon the foundation you build to achieve your goal. We all are goal oriented. We want results, that too easy and fast. We can conclude firmly that we Humans are very goal orientated. Trying to get slim and fit without settinga sure shot winning goal is almost like driving across a whole country without getting yourself a road map.It is simply a total waste of your precious time and money.It can even be even worse, you may never end up on your desired destination only.

The most important topic of concern initially will be that how do you set smart goals for yourself. Here we will be choosing the right kind of training partner.

If it is possible you must find the most reliable and a highly motivated training partner for yourself to follow the Badass Body Diet.

Choosing a partner will make things more interesting for you. It will provide you with another person to monitor and track your growth in terms of fitness. You will also have a partner to discuss all your weight loss achievements with.

It is very hard for most of us to ditch our commitments when there is another person involved into them. A good fitness workout partner will always help you and motivate you. You will specially need this partner when going gets really tough for you a good workout partner is a must. Well, the world's topnotch athletes, bodybuilders and competitors of various fitness competitions even always give creditsto their training partners for playing a vital role and being an integral part of their success. We are no different, so you must focus and pay attention on choosing the perfect companion for your own 6 week slim down challenge. It is definitely more worth it when you have a good support by your side to motivate you and keep you going in all times.

Now we are absolutely ready to start!

WEEK 1:
FIND AN EASY WAY FOR BETTER NUTRITION AND EXERCISE

One of the secrets of success of our Badass Body Diet 6 Weeks Slim Down is to pay keen attention to your pace. When you try to do all the things at once you wreck your whole regime before even really beginning it. The more efficient way to start is to improve your nutrition content and indulging yourself in better exercise and nutrition.

By following these tips, for you to stay motivated will be easy, but it will also help you to buildpositive momentum that will help you achieve weight loss you targeted for!

* Determine Your Own Fitness Level:-

To clearly understand where and how you are heading to, it is very important that the starting point makes ultimate sense. You must have a good understanding of how you approach your goal. You should not cheat with yourself and honestly analyze how in or how out of shape you are. Here are some things that can help you consider.

Counting the maximum number of push-ups you can do?

Keeping a close track of your own pulse before and your pulse after walking for a mile, your weight as well as your body fat percentage. Your level of endurance and strength will provide you a fair idea of how much exercise you can do in your first week without overdoing it or stressing yourself all in the first week.

* Start Walking More:-

On the three alternate days of your first week you must get moving by going for a brisk walk. This can be done anywhere like your neighborhood or at a nearby park or on a treadmill. Any which way you like. The duration of your walk must be based on how your body reacts to the 1 mile test. If by taking the test your pulse went really highthen you should start with 15 or 20 minutes ofinitial walking. If your pulse barely moved till the duration of 45 minutes. Remember and follow this goal for the 1st week. This way you can develop a habit of exercising regularly and you may also not end up being fully exhausted.

* Do Some Light Calisthenics:-

Calisthenics are simple exercises which help you tone your body muscles with the help of your ownbody weight. We will discuss about them in detail later, but as for now what we want is a light set of exercises just to start you up on those days where you are not walking.Three sets of push-ups on your kneesis fine, if you cannot do a full push-up,do ahalf of your maximum repetitions. Also with these bunch up three sets of as many sit ups or crunches you can do. All this is more than plenty for Week 1. You must remember to not to overdo it!

* Eliminate all Sugar Filled and Calorie Containing Drinks:-

A little diet adjustment can bring you back to the right track without you not even noticing it. All you have to do is cut drinking empty calories. You should Drop soda, also you should stop putting milk, cream and sugar to thetea or coffee you consume daily. You should replace these with water, coffee leaving the extras and green tea. You can also use stevia because it is a natural sweetener which is absolutely calorie free. These calorie sweeteners are substitutes to sugar. It will give you just the perfect taste of sugar but will not give you the calories that sugar has in it.

* Cut Out the Diet Busters:-

Week 1 is absolutely not about making the drastic changes in your diet, but it isabsolutely theright time to eliminate all your existing diet busters. You should completely stop consuming fast food, fried junk,candy and chips. Later we shall dig into strict concepts as well as methods related to diet. But for now you have to help you own self by eliminating all the junk food from your diet permanently.

I hope this 1st Week of our Badass Body Diet 6 Weeks Slim Down has not at all been tough. It isabout easing your way to be active and also eating right. By starting slow it will definitely help you build a concrete foundation for the weight loss goals that you will achieve if you are determined throughout. You don't have to worry. You just have to work hard and stay focused! I hope you are very excited about you own transformation!

You should certainly be very excited because a whole new transformation waits for you in the future!

WEEK:
2 SHOPPING GUIDELINES- HOW TO INTERPRET NUTRITION LABELS AND SHOP TO EAT BETTER

It is absolutely shocking that a lot of people follow a diet that burns fat without even investing little amount of time into doing some research about the food they eat. Apart from following the exercise program correctly you must also understand that a perfect diet will contribute to achieving your goal for that to achieve, you must know how to read and interpret nutrition labels on various food products. When you do not really know what is inside your food you will not be able to achieve what you really desire. When you understand the food labels correctly you will be able to shop better and eat better.

Let us now discuss what all does the nutrition label reveals about the product so that from further on you can certainly make wiser choices and eat better.

* Serving Size:-

One should pay total and complete attention to this written on the nutrition label of the product. Everything that will follow will apply to number of serving to be only 1. Food companies tend to often increase this number to exaggerate the amount of servings inside a product container. This will make the calorie content of the product seem lower. This is a devious trick used by various food companies to lure the consumers into buying their products by sabotaging their diet needs.

* Percentage of the Daily Value:-

The average calorie intake is 2000 caloriesin a day for an average active person. This details is based on a general rough guideline given the fact that it can easily vary in gender, age, activity level, weight, height etc.

* Calories:-

It is as it is self-explanatory that this is the number of calories that the product contains per serving.

* Fat:-

This is the total fat of your body. Further fats are classified into saturated fats, Monounsaturated fats, Trans fat and polyunsaturated fats. Both saturated fat and Trans fat should be avoided. Both Monounsaturated and Polyunsaturated fats carry some benefits. These healthier fats are found in olive oil and avocado.

* Cholesterol:-

It is suggested that you should keep your cholesterol intake below a certain 300mgs a day in order to avoid the risk of heart diseases. Below 150mgs a day can be an ideal target.

* Sodium:-

High amount of sodium intake will enable you to retain more water inside your body and that will make you weigh more. It is suggested to stay below 1500mgs a day for a healthy heart.You must keep an eye on the prepared food as they are loaded with high amount of sodium often.

* Carbohydrates:-

Carbohydrates are split into fiber which is said to be very good for health and sugar which is said to be very bad for health. You should aim for a low intake of carbs while you slim down so that things can go on in a much smoother way.

* Protein:-

Protein will be your best friend when you follow your guide. You should be aiming for around a .5 gram for every pound you weigh. When you are working out on a rigorous exercise routine you can aim more too. This is the most common source of calorie intake.

* Vitamins and Minerals:-

This includes both minerals and vitamins which are naturally present in food as well as anything that is artificially added by the manufacturer into any food product. We will be discussing in deep about the specific vitamins and minerals that you must be looking on our Badass body diet in detail later in our guide. As for now you should take care of the daily amount of ingredients recommended that the label reveals to you.

* Ingredients:-

These will be listed withthe amount that is contained in the product. This is also another area where some food companies will try ditch you with numbers.

Now you are fully equipped with the information that is needed for you to shop smart and be able to understand and correctly interpret the information given on the nutrition labels on food products.

While slimming down, you must value knowledge and pay attention to it.

WEEK 3:
EXERCISE DOES NOT ALWAYS HAVE TO BE AT THE GYM

To have a gym membership for ourselves is good for anyone. Gyms are filled up with plenty equipment, they are other people around you working out and also there are large number of distractions in the gym too. However, it is not practical to reach the gym and workout. I do know that from my personalexperience that there may even be many instances time and again where the option left to you is training at home. Life can certainly be like this.

I can certainly tell you this from experience that you can have an ideal training session outside of the gym as well and ease your way to slimming down. Following are some tips that will help you ease your way through the slimming down routine.

* Walk or may be Run:-

Depending completely on your own fitness level andathletic experience, walking or may be running is a perfect way to get rid of all the excess fat without spending a single penny. Also while adopting to this natural method you will not get bored out of the boring gym routine as well. You may require a little time to get used to it. Also your body may also take some time to react to this new method of slimming down but trust me it is the most hassle free and easiest method to burn that extra oodles of weight that you are carrying around without a reason.

* Do Push Ups:-

One will be shocked to see photos of people's bodies that have been developed by doing just a hundred push-ups every day. This does sound like a lot to do but if you do push-ups even for three days a week also then also you will see the number of Push-ups you ca do increase constantly. Push-ups will help you not only to develop your triceps and chest but also help you to tone your upper body. One more advantage is that is that rather than flaunting a really masculine body, flaunting just a fit body ca work just perfectly for a lot of us.

* Focus on Core Training:-

It is very easy to get a good and perfect ab related work-out routine just at home. I would prefer some sets of crunches clubbed with leg lifts for myself. Four sets of as many repetitions that you can do on the day of your push-ups, that for 3 days a week. We cannot expect to see our clear abdominal definition until we shed out some of our extra fat, but you get rid of the fat is you will see some concrete results, you may feel good about this core type of training.

* Consider Some Light Weight Lifting Exercise:-

A few dumbbellsare not a big investment but they are perfect regarding doing multiple sets of curls and sets of shoulder presses. It is not a necessary requirement, but it is good to have them with you so that you can equip home training with some variety. You should stick with three of each set of resistances that you can handle for 12 to 15 reps while you slim down this way.

* The Good Magic of Pull Ups:-

All of us do not have the strength to pull them of successfully when we start doing pull ups, but once we do start it can help you achieve a total transformation. Three sets of these on the days you are doing your other weight exercises the number of repetitions as your body allows you.

Now not being able to reach the gym will no longer be entertained as an excuse for not slimming down!

WEEK 4:
THE IMPORTANCE OF MACRONUTRIENTS

For week 4 of our Badass Body Diet 6 Weeks Slim Down, we are going to take another detailed look at diet. For our weight loss purpose we will be viewing the diets as basically being split up between two important categories. The first is the micronutrients - which includes vitamins and minerals, these are the things that we need in small quantities that don't carry much calories. Most of us are quite familiar with all the functions of micronutrients.

The second category of macronutrients are more important for our success – proteins, fats and carbohydrates. These three things are the ones that we require in large amounts to function and there are different ways in which how we manipulate them and that can mean the difference between 7 Week Slim Down success and its failure.

Let us look at all the three macronutrients:-

*** Protein:-**

Proteins are the building blocks of life and of our new lean bodies, which are absolutely essential to help us look and feel great. They are also required to speed up our recovery from hard workout sessions. Keeping our protein levels high will also bring us lots of other benefits like even keeping us more resistant little things like the common cold.

It is worth repeating that we should aim for .5 a gram of protein for every pound we weigh while easily slimming down.

Here are some common protein counts of food that you may enjoy: a 4 oz chicken breast has 36 grams of protein, a whole egg has 6 grams of protein, a glass of milk has 16 grams and most protein shakes contain 28 grams of protein in a serving.

If your protein levels are consistently low then you should be expecting slower strength gains, fatigue and possibly even can cause you an injury!

* Carbohydrates:-

Carbohydrates provide energy which comprise our diets. While the requirement of even a small amount contributes to the body to help it function efficiently, consuming excess of carbohydrates is definitely a spoiler and proves to be a death blow for people who are trying to follow a weight loss regime.

Theideal level of carbohydrates is almost around 30% part of your daily calorie needs. The rest splits up between proteins and healthy fats. This quantity should be lowered down for sure if you are facing difficulties shedding that extra body fat. The Sugary carbs and the things like white pasta, white rice and potatoes should not be a part of your regular diet.

* Fats:-

We come on to fats. I wish to clear one of the most common misconceptions related to diet for once. All fats don't make you fat. As a matter of fact many are healthy and also work as weight loss miracles. Fish oil, flax seed oil and unsaturated fats of lesser degree (like olive oil) are important. Without them your diet is incomplete.

You should take 3 grams of flax or fish oil once in a day and then you should be prepared to see yourself lose weight faster.This will happen as your metabolism increases and the overall quality of your life will definitely improve. Inflammation will definitely decrease. In addition to this your skin and your hair will look great. Also many guys will experience increase in their sex drive! There is hardly anyother addition that you could have made in your diet which proves to be so transformative!

These tips will quickly start giving resultsin the favor of your slimming down process. Dieting can prove to be an effective method without getting complicated. When you apply these principles in Week 4 and beyond you will quickly see good results.

WEEK 5:
THE BENEFITS OF HIIT- The HIGH INTENSITY TRAINING WITH INTERVALS

What if I told you that instead of your monotonous gym routine, there is a super and fun way to charge up you cardio routine, and this way can definitely help you lose oodles of fat in just little bit of time as compared to the traditional workout methods? Well there certainly is a way to do it. It is called asHigh Intensity Training with Intervals (HITI) and this is the main focus of the Week five of our whole slim down process. So now you should be prepared to sweat it out!

What do you mean byHigh Intensity Training with Intervals?

High Intensity Training with Intervals is an exercise technique that contains short ways of near to maximum or maximum strength cardio routine with little exertion or low intensity periods. Every segment can differently vary.

This is what a common HITI routine looks like:-

It is around of 2 minute intensive running and 3 minutes of normal jogging will follow it. You should do around 4 rounds for that. The Total Cardio HITI Workout time is equal to 20 minutes. This method can burn to about four times the calories that are burned by an average intensity 45 minutes of cardio session!

Benefits of HITI:-

Here is a detailed look at some of the advantages of HITI training that is enough to inspire you to leave all the old school cardio routines for good.

* HITI destroys Your Body Fat:-

We are looking to become Slim and thereforethe benefit of HITIis dearest to us. HITI burns off excess fat in a very fewer time but it also getsthis – it increasesthe metabolic state and your body burns calories for many hours even after the workout routine is over. That will work remarkably well for your slimming down process.

* HITI Builds Your Muscles along with Cutting on Fats:-

A remarkable feature of HITI is that it works well to preserve the hard earned muscles alongside torching your fat. Have you ever noticed the difference between a normal Olympic marathon runner's thin body and an Olympic sprinter's perfectly toned plus amazing looking physique? This is so because the marathon athletes use old cardio methods for their training purpose while the sprinters often use HITI drills!

* HITI is the most Efficient for Building Endurance:-

Many Studies and researches have suggested that HITI training builds stamina amazingly fast and in a more efficient way than other long bouts of low intensity cardio. It does Sound counter instinctive but the facts and science in the researches are very clear about it. HITI wins the race by miles.

* HITIalso Improves the Insulin Sensitivity:-

HITI carves your body highly to be responsive to insulin, this results to fewer body fats getting accumulated throughout your daily routines. This benefit can be felt also on the days you perform the HITI, but it even carries for a week.

* HITI Develops the body Energy Systems:-

The HITI training helps to develop your anaerobic and aerobic energy systems both. This en cashes to a splendid performance in a short time span. HITI cardio proficiency will add repetitions to all the other exercises that are done at the gymnasium. The various forms of cardio do not affect your anaerobic systems.

For the 5th Week and after that my suggestion would be to shift your cardio workout days to HITI sessions. You can use this workout above for 3 days in a week, and then you will be able to see the amazing and dramatic changes in yourself.

WEEK 6:
TRANSFORM THIS DIET INTO A LIFESTYLE AND NOT ONLY 6 WEEKS

There is absolutely no doubtthat with the help of hard work, motivation, self-Discipline and aworkout program like this onewill make you achieve incredible changes to your body. I have personally seen people transform into completely new versions of themselves for better and for good.

Real and long lasting change is achieved when you adopt a new lifestyle and notonly a new program.

The methods mentioned in this guide are all safe and effective and I hope that they inspire you to adopt the foundation of a whole new fit, slim and healthy way of living.

Here are some ideas that will help you achieve a fit and healthy lifestyle in record time. Enjoy Yourself!

* Never Break the Three Law:-

Commit with yourself to follow the cardio regime for at least 3 days, may it be HITI or not, and at least 3 days of weight training or resistance training. Cardio and strength training can be done on the same day if there any issue pertaining to time. But you must never break the three law unless you are deathly ill.

* Stick to A Healthy Diet:-

You must keep your momentum of sticking to a healthy diet going. An Occasional cheat day is fine, but be careful and avoid eating all the junk food that comes in your way. Keeping your diet clean is a must otherwise you will need another 6 Week Slim Down after some time.

* Make Fit Friends:-

Positive peer pressure will always be a wonderful motivation. With fit friends around you, you will feel the urge to keep moving in the direction of being healthy

* Explore New Exciting Fitness Activities:-

Why not explore yoga, Pilates or the fun and craziness of Kettlebell conditioning? Fresh and new fitness experiences can also help in motivating you and it will definitely help you have an athletic figure.

* Teach What You Have Learned:-

Sharing your experiences is a great way to move in the right direction.

I hope the idea and the thought of staying fit for life makes you feel excited. There cannot be a better way of achieving life's challenges than being slim, strong, looking great and with a smile on your face. The alternative is not that appealing for sure.

CONCLUSION:
NOW IS THE TIME TO CHANGE YOUR LIFE

If you are feeling tired and slow, you can't fit into your own clothes, you just can't see yourself going out of shape, you see yourself having health and weight related issues. This is the time where you should seriously consider of introducing yourself to some change in your life.

You might want to back out and give yourselves a lot of excuses, but then you have to make your will strong and continue to change yourself.

This is the high time when you should completely change your life.

I would like to present just a few more thoughts on the subject.

* Putting off your goals will be the quickest path to kill them. When you don't take positive action towards your goals, you will be letting your goals die.

* Accept Responsibility. If you really want to bring change and transform your life, you should accept the responsibility for everything and try and change it on your own. Nobody but you have to do it.

* Be Willing and Ready To Make Change. It is a great start. When you keep that positive outlook

throughout the 6 weeks it will let you achieve greater heights.

* Ignore your Limitations. Most of the limitations are creations that we ourselves construct in our minds. When you follow our guide with a positive mind and attitude you will achieve the impossible

Do not hesitate to bring change in your life, because this is the right time to do it.

Thank you and good luck!

WaraWaran Roongruangsri